Natalika Kraft

My Guide – Dementia

Tips for Family and Friends
- concise and to the point -

Table of Contents

Familiar Environment or Nursing Home?	3
Home Design	5
Choosing Colors for Home Design	10
Communication	13
Aggression	17
Leisure Activities	19
Experience Togetherness	21
Interaction	22
Urge to Move	25
The Animals	28
Nutrition	30
Food Refusal	34
What Makes People with Dementia Happy?	36
Conclusion	38
IMPRINT	39

Familiar Environment or Nursing Home?

The decision between maintaining the familiar environment and opting for a nursing home for a person with dementia is often complex and depends on various factors. Here are some considerations:

Familiar Environment

Familiarity and Security: The familiar environment can provide a sense of security and familiarity, which is particularly important for people with dementia. Preservation of Routines: Maintaining familiar routines and habits can help reduce anxieties and confusion.

Support from Family Members: If caregiving family members are present and supportive services are available, home care can be a good option. Personalized Care: Individualized care tailored to the specific needs of the person can be more easily provided in the home environment.

Nursing Home

Professional Care: Nursing homes often provide professional care around the clock, including medical support that may not be available at home.
Social Interaction: Nursing homes frequently facilitate more social interactions and activities, which can be crucial for emotional well-being.

Safety Measures: Nursing homes are typically designed to create a safe environment for people with dementia, with specialized safety measures in place.
Relief for Family Members: Providing care at home can impose a high burden on family members. A nursing home can offer relief and provide opportunities for breaks.

It is important to note that the decision should be made individually and depends on specific needs, financial resources, and support from family and friends. Often, a combination of home care and professional support is a good solution.
Thorough evaluation of the individual situation, consultation with dementia care professionals, and open discussions with the affected person and their family members can help in decision-making. It is essential to respect the needs and wishes of the person with dementia, where possible, and ensure the best possible support.

Home Design

The design of the everyday environment plays a crucial role in caring for individuals with memory loss. Here are some tips for home design for caregivers of dementia patients:

Reducing Overstimulation:
Remove unnecessary items and decorations to create a calm and clutter-free environment.
Avoid bright colors and complex patterns to minimize visual distractions.

Orientation Aids:
Use clear and prominently visible labels for doors, rooms, and important areas.
Set up prominent landmarks or memory cues to aid orientation.

Safety Measures:
Remove potentially dangerous items such as sharp tools or toxic substances.
Install safety features like non-slip rugs and handrails.

Comfortable and Familiar Furniture:
Arrange furniture in a logical layout and create clear pathways through the rooms.

Use familiar furniture pieces to foster a sense of familiarity and security.

Memorabilia and Photos:
Incorporate personal memorabilia and photos to promote positive memories.
Create a photo wall with pictures of family, friends, and important events.

Lighting Design:
Ensure adequate lighting, especially in hallways, stairs, and other potential tripping hazards.
Utilize natural light to support the day-night rhythm.

Flexible Use of Spaces:
Allow for flexible use of spaces to enable the affected individual to move freely.
Consider different needs, such as quiet areas for retreat.

Communication Aids:
Place important information in writing, such as a bulletin board for appointments or messages.
Use clear and simple language in communication.

Regular Activities:
Set up regular activity areas that align with the interests of the individual.

Provide opportunities to participate in light household chores or hobbies.

Flexible Adjustments:
Monitor the progression of the illness and adapt home design flexibly to changing needs.
Individual needs may vary, so it's important to address the specific requirements and preferences of the dementia patient. Seeking professional advice from experts in dementia care could also be helpful.

Hazard Minimization:
Conceal electrical cords and remove loose carpets to minimize tripping hazards. Install Childproofing on

Outlets and Sharp Corners:
Install childproofing devices on outlets and sharp corners to prevent accidents.

Quiet Environment:
Minimize loud noises and create a calm environment to reduce stress and confusion.
Use curtains or carpets to absorb sound.

Accessible Design:
Ensure that the home is accessible to facilitate easier movement.
Consider using ramps or elevators to overcome height differences.

Kitchen Adaptations:
Simplify the kitchen by providing only necessary utensils and dishes.
Mark switches and knobs for easy visibility.

Supporting Daily Routine:
Establish a structured daily routine with fixed meal times and rest periods.
Use clocks or calendars to organize the day.

Technological Aids:
Utilize technology such as doorbell cameras or GPS trackers to enhance safety.
Install simple digital clocks or calendars with reminder functions.

Flexible Furniture:
Use easily movable furniture to adapt room configuration to needs.
Consider height-adjustable beds and chairs for comfortable use.

Calming Elements:
Integrate calming elements like indoor plants or aquariums to create a relaxed atmosphere.
Explore the possibility of aromatherapy with pleasant scents.

Simple Toilet Design:
Ensure the bathroom is easily accessible and equipped with non-slip mats.
Install grab bars near the toilet and in the shower.

Professional Consultation:
Consult a dementia care expert or interior designer for tailored recommendations.
Learn about local support services and resources for dementia care.

The home design should aim to create a safe, comfortable, and supportive environment that meets the individual needs of the dementia patient. It can also be helpful to make regular adjustments to accommodate changing abilities and challenges.

Choosing Colors for Home Design

When selecting colors for home design for individuals with dementia, there are several principles to consider that can help create a positive and supportive environment. Here are some general considerations:

Soothing Colors:
Soft and calming tones such as pastels, gentle blues and greens, and earth tones can create a relaxed atmosphere.
These colors can help reduce stress and promote a peaceful environment.

Contrast for Visibility:
Adequate contrast between walls, furniture, and flooring aids visibility and object differentiation.
For instance, use darker colors for furniture against a lighter wall.

Color Consistency:
Consistent color scheme throughout the home can minimize confusion and facilitate clear orientation.
Avoid too many different colors in one room.

Avoidance of Excessive Patterns:
Reduce complex patterns as they can confuse. Uniform colors and simple patterns are often more suitable.

Bright Colors for Lighting:
Bright wall colors and ceilings can better reflect light and ensure a well-lit environment.
Good lighting is essential to minimize uncertainties in the room.

Personalized Accents:
Integrate personal touches in the individual's preferred colors to create a familiar and positive environment. Photos, artworks, or decorations in favorite colors can foster a positive mood.

Avoidance of Red:
Red hues may exacerbate agitation or restlessness in some individuals with dementia.
It's recommended to steer clear of intense red tones.

Nature-inspired Colors:
Colors reflecting elements of nature, such as green for plants or blue for water, can have a calming effect. Nature-inspired colors can evoke positive associations.

It's important to note that individual preferences and sensitivities may vary. It could be helpful to observe the individual's reaction to specific colors and adjust accordingly. In any case, it's advisable to align home design with the individual needs and preferences of the person with dementia.

Communication

Individuals with Alzheimer's or another form of dementia gradually lose their ability to communicate verbally, which can be painful for all involved. Normal conversations with a mother or father, partner, or spouse become difficult and eventually impossible. It is important to repeatedly put oneself in the position of the affected person and adapt one's own way of communication according to their current understanding. Through experimentation and with some luck, ways can be found to stay in conversation or at least in emotional contact with each other.

Nonverbal communication plays a central role in dealing with people with dementia. Most of them retain mastery of body language longer than verbal communication. With increasing difficulties in verbal communication, they tend to express their messages through gestures and pointing. At the same time, they are particularly attentive to our body language. This presents both opportunities and unexpected challenges.

To help them better understand content messages, we can supplement our words with gestural and pantomimic elements. This can be particularly helpful, for example, when giving instructions for personal care or asking for assistance in household tasks.

Some emotional messages can also be conveyed without words. Touches such as stroking, hugging, or giving a massage are immediate ways of communication. Physical affection can often create a deeper connection than any spoken word. However, it is always important to consider whether the affected person actually desires physical closeness.

Memory aids are important. As long as dementia has not taken away the ability of the individual to understand written information, small notes with information about daily routines or answers to frequently asked questions can be helpful. These notes can be placed, for example, on the refrigerator or bathroom door, allowing them to be read in passing. A "family poster" with photos of all household members can also support people with dementia. Each photo is accompanied by brief information, including about household aids, caregivers, and even pets.

Since many important events fade from awareness during the course of dementia, a memory book can be helpful. Create a photo album that recalls beautiful moments. Write a short sentence for each photo, such as what event it is, who is depicted, and perhaps a little anecdote. It's not about capturing as many milestones as possible, but those that are particularly meaningful to the person with dementia. With the memory book, you create a foundation for communication, both for yourself and for caregivers.

Important Communication Rules for Interacting with People with Dementia:

- Establish eye contact at their eye level before each conversation and address people with dementia by their name.
- Use the local dialect when speaking with dialect speakers if possible, to build trust and improve communication.
- Avoid technical jargon, slang, and complicated multisyllabic terms, especially when comprehension difficulties exist.
- Speak slightly slower and clearly. Use short sentences.
- Frame questions in a way that can be answered with a single word or with yes/no, especially for straightforward information exchange.
- Offer no more than two options at once, especially in later stages of dementia.
- Allow people with dementia sufficient time and peace for responses. Pauses between sentences are important.

- Repeat important information and utilize positive keywords.
- Avoid irony, metaphorical meanings, and negative phrasing. Express messages positively.
- Consider that people with dementia often take language literally. Use clear and understandable expressions.
- Pose questions that the affected person can answer, particularly regarding feelings, perceptions, or opinions.
- Acknowledge and praise good performance. Do not criticize for mistakes.
- Overlook peculiar expressions or incorrect words without comment. Avoid corrections.
- Steer clear of arguments, insistence on being right, and confronting with misplaced items.
- Ignore accusations and reproaches; respond with empathy and change the subject.
- Recognize that sometimes less is more, and accept shared silence if it is perceived as comforting.
- It is important to adjust communication to the current understanding of the person with dementia and adapt accordingly during conversations.

Aggression

It is important to understand that unfriendly or aggressive behavior in people with dementia often stems from factors related to the disease. Here are some reasons for such behavior and approaches to handle it:

Understanding the Disease:
People with dementia can feel lost in their environment and may not properly assess situations. A lack of understanding of what is happening around them can lead to frustration and aggression.

Communication Problems:
As dementia progresses, verbal communication becomes challenging. People with dementia may struggle to express themselves adequately, leading to frustration and aggression.

Changes in Personality:
The personality of people with dementia can change throughout the course of the disease. This can lead to conflicts, especially if old family issues resurface.

Seeking Outside Help:
Family members and caregivers may reach their limits when dealing with aggressive behavior. In such cases,

seeking professional help from outside sources can be beneficial to avoid conflicts and respond appropriately.

Maintaining Calm:
It is important to remain calm in such situations. A calm and empathetic approach can help calm the person's mood and minimize conflicts.

Professional Support:
A dementia care expert or psychologist can offer valuable advice and strategies for dealing with aggressive behavior. Sometimes, specialized care facilities may be necessary.

It is crucial to understand that aggressive reactions are often a result of the disease itself and should not be perceived as a personal attack. An empathetic and supportive approach can help improve the quality of life for people with dementia and their caregivers.

Leisure Activities

It is common for many people with dementia to give up their leisure activities, driven by fear of judgment from others and their own fear of failure. However, as someone affected by dementia, it is advisable to maintain hobbies and interests for as long as possible and to stay active. This helps to preserve cognitive function for longer and maintain a sense of balance.

It is important not to give up hobbies but to adapt them to current circumstances! Some people enjoy singing and dancing, while others regularly bowl or hike. Even after a dementia diagnosis, you should try to continue your favorite activities for as long as possible. Song lyrics, dance steps, and movement patterns often remain in memory longer.

By continuing activities, you can retain what you have learned for longer and at the same time train your independence. If familiar activities, such as dancing, don't work as well anymore, you can simplify the steps, move freely to the music, or sway. If orienteering becomes difficult, there is always the option to hike or take walks with others.

It is also advisable to try out new activities to find out what brings you joy. Perhaps you would like to participate in a birdwatching tour, take a comedy or theater course, paint, or drum. In the course of dementia, many people discover surprisingly new aspects of themselves and often find new interests that they enthusiastically devote themselves to by chance.

However, when trying out new activities, do not overexert yourself. Less, but more calmly performed activities are often better. The most important thing is to stay active and have fun!

Experience Togetherness

Friends and family may not always have time to fulfill all your social needs. However, organized group activities can provide you with many opportunities and variety. In church communities, sports clubs, and cultural groups, you can meet like-minded people. In groups with other affected individuals, you can experience mutual understanding and support.

In the advanced stages of dementia, you can join others in day care centers for activities such as games, singing, or simply having coffee together. You can obtain information about groups in your area from organizations such as the German Alzheimer's Society or a welfare association.

It is helpful to create a daily schedule. Structure your day so that there are fixed times for all activities such as sleeping, eating, and washing. Your leisure activities such as reading the newspaper, taking walks, or meeting with others should also be firmly anchored in this schedule. This way, you maintain orientation and avoid unnecessary stress.

Interaction

Interacting with people suffering from dementia plays a crucial role in promoting their mental activity while also achieving much-needed relief from dementia symptoms. Games specifically designed for dementia patients offer an exciting and mentally stimulating avenue. Through such games, individuals can engage in meaningful activities and train their memory in everyday life. Additionally, these games contribute to increasing overall well-being, promoting joy, and even strengthening communication skills.

Selecting games for people with dementia requires simple, easily understandable options that promote enjoyment, entertainment, and mental activity.

Here are some types of games that may be considered suitable:

Board games and card games:
Games such as Memory, Dominoes, Bingo, or simple card games with large cards can stimulate cognitive function.
Ensure that the rules of the game are simple, and the game can be played in a short amount of time.

Puzzles and shape games:
Large puzzle pieces with simple pictures or shapes can promote hand-eye coordination and spatial perception. Wooden puzzles with handles may be particularly well-suited.

Word games:
Crossword puzzles with simple words or word search puzzles can promote language skills.
Word games can also be presented in the form of cards or magnetic letters.

Music and memory games:
Games associated with music, such as guessing songs or matching musical instruments, can be enjoyable. Memory games related to personal stories or events can stimulate positive conversations.

Movement games:
Simple movement games such as seated dancing, ball games, or target throwing can improve motor skills and encourage activity.
Take into account physical limitations and adjust activities accordingly.

Digital games for seniors:
There are specialized apps and games designed for seniors that can be played on tablets or simple consoles.

Such games can provide cognitive challenges and promote the use of technology.

Creative games:
Creative activities such as painting, crafting, or simple handicrafts can have a positive and calming effect.
Use easily manageable materials and encourage artistic expression.

Simulation games:
Games that simulate activities from daily life, such as gardening, kitchen activities, or household tasks, can evoke memories.
They can serve as conversation starters and address practical skills.

When selecting games, it is important to consider the individual preferences and abilities of the person with dementia. Observe reactions and adjust the games as needed to provide a positive and enriching experience.

Urge to Move

The urge to move in people with dementia is not fundamentally negative, as it can promote balance, muscle tone, and circulation. However, associated behaviors can be problematic. In care facilities, conflicts with fellow residents may arise when affected individuals constantly enter their rooms. Additionally, there are dangers such as leaving the premises unaccompanied due to impaired orientation.

Another risk is that some individuals with dementia continue to walk despite exhaustion, leading to significant weight loss even if they regularly eat meals. The physical exertion of walking can also result in hypoglycemia, with behavioral issues similar to those of diabetics.

However, the greatest problem lies in the danger of falls and fractures due to incessant wandering. It is therefore important to take appropriate safety measures and monitor the movement activities of people with dementia to minimize potential risks. There are various ways to address the urge to move in people with dementia and minimize potential dangers:

Medical Examination: Pain or illnesses such as urinary tract infections could be causes for constant wandering. A medical examination can help rule out such causes.

Safety Measures: Remove tripping hazards, install handrails in the home, and wear sturdy shoes to prevent falls.

Calorie-rich Snacks: Providing juices, small fruit plates, and other calorie-rich treats along usual walking paths to minimize weight loss and hypoglycemia.

Positive Approach: Individuals with a strong urge to move should be greeted positively and invited to sit on the sofa rather than reacting with misunderstanding or anger.

Securing the Front Door: For those who are disoriented, the front door can be secured with an alarm to prevent unnoticed exits.

Shared Gardens in Care Facilities: Large, fenced gardens allow individuals with dementia to move freely and safely.

Group Walks: Daily walks of at least 30 minutes in the surroundings can be offered.

Structured Activities: Regular activities like chair dancing, senior gymnastics, communal singing, or biographically anchored tasks can interrupt the urge to move.

Emotional Stimulation: Distraction through favorite music, religious services, or interactions with children and pets can encourage individuals with dementia to sit longer.

Swinging: The use of a safe rehabilitation rocking chair can help dissipate nervous energy.

Comfortable Environment: Lighting, tranquility, and comfortable seating can help individuals with dementia stay longer.

Location Systems: The use of location systems such as GPS trackers is ethically controversial but is advocated by some caregivers.

The Animals

The reaction of people with dementia to animals can vary greatly, but many experience positive effects in their presence.

Here are some general observations

Calmness and Stress Reduction:
Animals, especially dogs and cats, can have a calming effect and reduce stress. The soft touch and fur of animals can provide a soothing sensory experience.

Promotion of Social Interactions:
Animals can promote social interactions and trigger positive emotions. Taking care of a pet can provide a meaningful task and instill a sense of responsibility.

Memories and Conversation Stimulation:
Animals can evoke positive memories and stimulate conversations about past pets or experiences. Sharing stories about animals can lead to positive interactions.

Increase in Physical Activity:
The presence of animals can encourage movement, whether through walks with a dog or playing with a cat. Physical activity can improve well-being and mood.

Reduction of Isolation:
Pets can reduce loneliness and social isolation by providing companionship. The emotional connection to an animal can provide a sense of connection.

Improvement of Quality of Life:
Studies show that the presence of animals can improve the quality of life for people with dementia. Animal-assisted interventions are also used in care facilities to promote the well-being of residents.

It is important to note that not all people with dementia react positively to animals. Some may develop fears or uncertainties about animals, especially if they have not had pets before or have had negative experiences. In such cases, it is important to respect the person's reactions and seek alternative approaches to promoting well-being.

Before introducing a pet into the environment of a person with dementia, it is advisable to consider individual preferences, past experiences, and any potential allergic reactions. Visits from specially trained therapy animals can also enable positive interaction without requiring a permanent commitment.

Nutrition

People living with Alzheimer's or another form of dementia struggle not only with memory problems; often, their sense of taste diminishes, and the sensation of hunger and thirst diminishes as well. To prevent physical weakness and nutritional deterioration associated with dementia, people with dementia need to maintain a balanced diet and drink enough fluids. Regular meal times can help support this.

Certain foods promote brain health.
We can actively influence our mental quickness and brain fitness, among other things, through a balanced and healthy diet.

There is no single food that optimizes and maintains our mental fitness permanently. However, studies show that a diet with specific foods can indeed help preserve our cognitive abilities in the long term. It is advisable to start as early as possible.

A study at the German Center for Neurodegenerative Diseases (DZNE) examined the effects of a Mediterranean diet rich in fruits, vegetables, legumes, olive oil, and regular consumption of fatty fish. In this study, 512 participants were surveyed about their dietary habits. Cognitive abilities, such as memory, were examined, as were the presence of specific proteins in the cerebrospinal fluid. Researchers looked for proteins that cause deposits and cell adhesions, which are in turn associated with the development of Alzheimer's disease.

The result of the study shows that those who followed a Mediterranean diet – consuming lots of vegetables, fruits, and fatty fish – not only performed better in memory tests but also
had fewer of the suspicious proteins in their bodies.

A separate study from 2018 showed that consuming one serving of green leafy vegetables such as spinach, kale, or chard daily can measurably slow down brain aging. Particularly, the nutrients folate (folic acid), lutein (a yellow plant pigment commonly found in green leafy vegetables), and phylloquinone or vitamin K1 were responsible for this effect, according to the researchers.

However, it is important to note that our brains also require energy, which it obtains from carbohydrates. Complex carbohydrates are optimal. Daniela Krehl, a nutritionist at the Consumer Center of Bavaria, emphasizes: "The brain cannot derive energy from fat or protein; therefore, one should regularly consume complex carbohydrates, such as whole grain pasta, whole grain bread, brown rice, or potatoes."

Furthermore, our brains require adequate fluid intake, as a lack thereof can lead to concentration difficulties and headaches. Krehl warns: "It is very important for mental fitness to drink enough fluids. A fluid loss of just two percent can lead to difficulties in concentration and headaches. One and a half liters per day are definitely advisable."

The following foods are considered beneficial for the brain:

- Green leafy vegetables such as spinach, chard, kale, pak choi, and savoy cabbage
- Olive oil and other healthy, cold-pressed oils like rapeseed oil, flaxseed oil, or walnut oil
- Nuts such as walnuts, almonds, cashews, hazelnuts, and pistachios
- Fatty fish like herring, salmon, and mackerel
- Fiber-rich carbohydrates found in whole grain bread, potatoes, oatmeal, whole grain pasta, brown rice, and in legumes such as lentils or beans
- Turmeric
- Foods with antioxidant properties such as green tea or beetroot

- Berries like blueberries, strawberries, and raspberries
- Low-sugar fruits
- Coffee or caffeine in moderation
- Use of iodized salt

To ensure that people with dementia do not forget to eat, it is advisable to maintain regular meal times. These set times for breakfast, lunch, and dinner can be recorded on a schedule. Such a visual overview can be particularly helpful for individuals who can still read, to structure their days and not neglect eating.

For individuals with dementia living alone, external support can be especially useful. Although nowadays mobile apps can be used as reminders for meals, it may be more motivating if, for example, children or friends call regularly to remind about the next meal. A "Meals on Wheels" service provided by a welfare organization can also ensure some regularity, at least once a day. If eating alone doesn't bring joy, organizing a volunteer visiting service could be considered. A volunteer could then occasionally eat together with the affected person.

Food Refusal

During dementia, food refusal can occur for various reasons. Firstly, toothaches, ill-fitting dentures, or inflammation in the oral cavity can lead to rejection of food. If the affected person grimaces in pain while eating or repeatedly interrupts the eating process, it is advisable to promptly consult a dentist.

Secondly, in the advanced stages of dementia, due to the slowed closing of the epiglottis during swallowing, the person may occasionally choke and then cough vigorously to remove the food bolus from the airways.

This can be perceived as extremely frightening and life-threatening, so even people with advanced dementia may prefer to refrain from eating out of fear of choking. Once such swallowing difficulties occur, speech therapy treatment should be prescribed by the attending physician. In such swallowing therapy, correct posture during eating and drinking is practiced, and focus is placed on chewing and swallowing. Additionally, caregivers are taught that food intake can be improved and facilitated by various forms of thickened food.

Thirdly, depression can also lead to food refusal. While food intake is important, one should never attempt to force a person with dementia to eat.

Food and drinks should always be offered without pressure. The question of whether and when artificial nutrition in the form of a PEG tube (percutaneous endoscopic gastrostomy) is advisable must be decided on an individual basis. The presumed will of the person with dementia should be taken into account in this decision.

What Makes People with Dementia Happy?

Numerous aspects can contribute to people with dementia experiencing happiness in their daily lives. Firstly, it is crucial to spend time with friends and family to create a sense of love and connection.

However, what is particularly important is recognizing what brings joy specifically to someone with dementia and understanding their individual needs and preferences. Since people with dementia have different interests, there are diverse ways to experience happiness. Therefore, caregivers and family members need to discover which activities best suit each individual.

For some people, physical activities such as walks or dancing can brighten their mood and create joyful moments. Others with dementia may enjoy activities like art, music, or games to experience happiness.

The caregiving staff needs to consider the changing needs of the person over time and ensure their participation in meaningful activities that bring joy.

By providing meaningful activities in their environment, people with dementia have the opportunity to enjoy life while dealing with their illness.

Conclusion

Experiencing happiness in people with dementia can indeed be multifaceted and individual. Even as their ability for verbal communication diminishes, they can continue to experience joy and contentment.

It is important to consider the individual preferences and needs of the person with dementia. Compassionate and attentive care can help create moments of happiness and improve their quality of life.

****

I create my books with the greatest love and care. However, errors are not always avoidable. If your copy has any defects, such as faulty binding or printing errors, please contact the platform through which you purchased the book to receive a replacement.

For further concerns, I am available via email at:
Lik.Verlag@gmail.com

If you enjoyed this book, I would greatly appreciate a review on Amazon. Your positive review can help me tremendously. Thank you for your support!

IMPRINT

Natalika Kraft is represented by:

Natalya Cernov
Thüringer Str. 47
73207 Plochingen
Lik.Verlag@gmail.com

The information and advice in this book have been carefully checked by the author, but no guarantee is provided. The author and publisher cannot be held liable for any errors or potential damages. This work is protected by copyright, and reproduction and distribution, except for private, non-commercial purposes, are prohibited and will be prosecuted under civil and criminal law. This applies particularly to the distribution of the work through photocopies, film, radio and television, electronic media, and the internet, as well as for commercial use of recipes, instructions, or similar content.

Designed by LikVerlag
Copyright © LikVerlag 2024 – All rights reserved

www.ingramcontent.com/pod-product-compliance
Lightning Source LLC
Chambersburg PA
CBHW071202240526
45470CB00017B/1230